YOUR HEADACHE
ISN'T ALL IN YOUR HEAD

Neuroscience Education for
Patients with Headache Pain

Adriaan Louw
PT, PhD, CSMT

Ina Diener
PT, PhD

ISBN #978-0-9857186-6-4

Index

SCIENTIFIC SUPPORT FOR YOUR RECOVERY

In each section, you will notice some numbers in the sentences. These numbers refer to scientific articles that support the statements in your book. The details of each article are listed at the back of your book.

The author of the book would like to offer special thanks to the artist, Rod Bohner, and the editor, Carolyn Raymond.

Understanding Your Pain

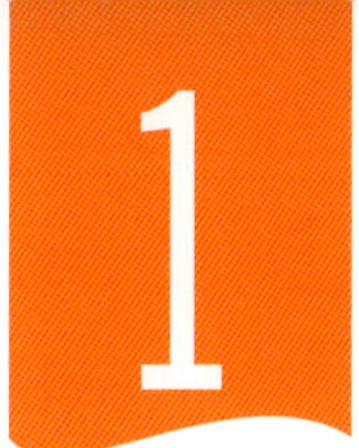

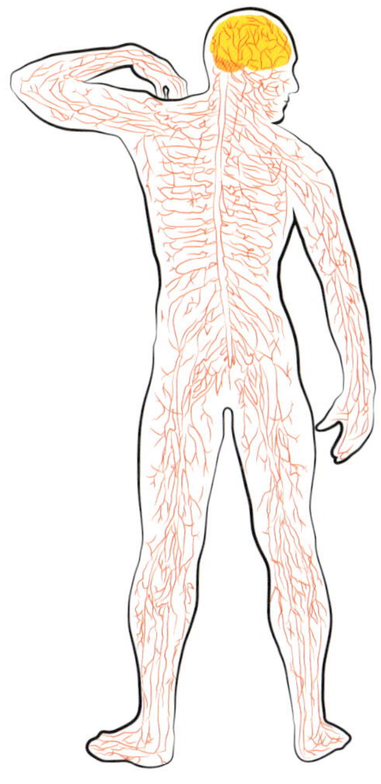

Pain is a normal human experience.[1] Without the ability to experience pain, humans would not survive. Learning about how pain works will help you understand why you hurt.

In your body, as well as in the bodies of all humans, there are over 400 individual nerves. Think about 45 miles of nerves traveling through the body and connecting all body parts. These nerves are all connected like a highway system.[2]

Nerves work like an alarm system. At all times, nerves have a small amount of electricity traveling through them. This is normal and shows you're alive. The nerves' activity increases or decreases depending on many factors in your life such as stress, movement, and temperature.

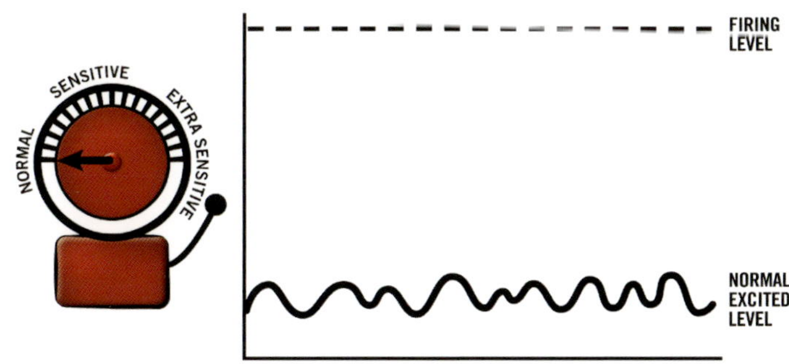

Although nerves are affected by many factors, they do have thresholds. When nerves become excited enough to reach the threshold, the message from the area will be sent on to your brain for analysis and appropriate action. For example, if you step on a rusted nail, do you want to know about it? Of course you do. You'll want to take the nail out, get a tetanus shot, protect your injured foot and give it time to heal.[3]

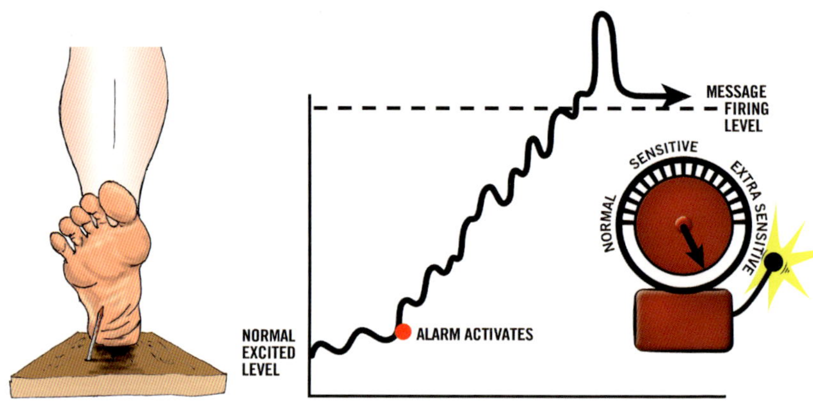

As soon as the alarm goes off and sends the message, the alarm system will return to its resting level, ready to warn you of additional danger. In the rusted nail example, the message travels from the foot to the spinal cord to the brain. It alerts the brain there is something going on and to take action. In this case, the action is that the brain produces pain to alert you that your injured foot needs attention. The pain prompts the additional action of getting the nail removed.

Pain is 100% produced by your brain. It's produced when the brain believes you are under threat and need protection.[4] As an example, think about an ankle sprain. If you sprained your ankle right now, would it hurt? Undoubtedly, you would answer "yes" because an ankle injury is associated with pain. But what happens if you sprain your ankle while crossing a busy street? As you roll your ankle, you see a speeding bus heading straight for you. It's not stopping. Does the ankle still hurt? Of course not! In this case, it isn't logical for the brain to produce pain in the ankle because pain in the ankle would cause you to fall down, grab the ankle and be hit by the speeding bus. If you could listen in on the brain during that decision-making situation, the brain would have to decide if a speeding bus is more dangerous than an ankle sprain. Because the bus is

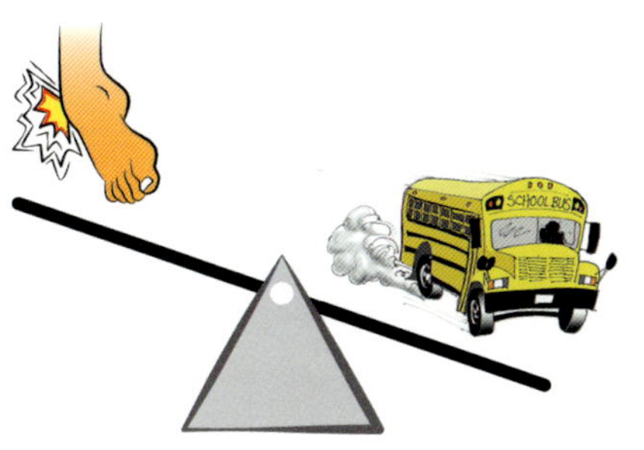

obviously more dangerous, pain is not produced in the ankle and you run out of the way. After the bus speeds by, the brain may decide to produce pain in the ankle to alert you to get treatment for your ankle sprain.

Tissue injury and pain are two different things. You can have pain, but no tissue injury. You can have an injury, but no pain. For example, have you ever noticed blood on your body or a scrape or bruise and had no idea where it came from? In this case, you had a tissue injury, but no pain was produced. Tissues constantly send information to the brain. In some cases, the brain produces pain to get your attention, slow you down and force you to take care of the issue. In some cases, it doesn't. **The good news is that pain does not necessarily indicate that there is something wrong in the tissues.**

Understanding Your Headache

Headaches can seem complex and confusing. When you consider the numerous doctor visits and medical tests, the frustration of failed treatments, the negative impact on your life and the persistent pain, it's no wonder headaches seem not only complex, but also confusing.

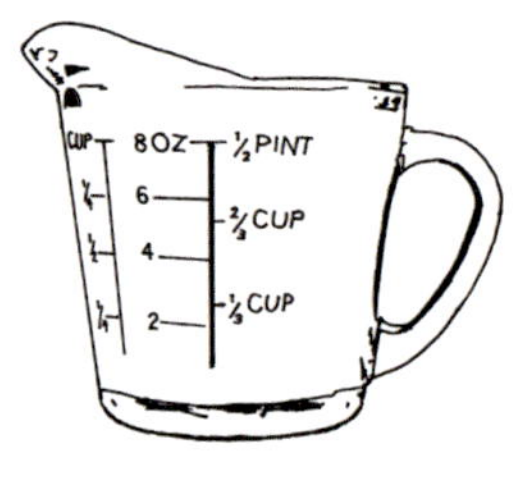

Here's a simple image that can help you understand headaches. Think about an empty measuring cup. If water is continually poured into the cup, it will overflow. If you can grasp this idea, you are well on your way to understanding your headaches and understanding why certain treatments may help you.

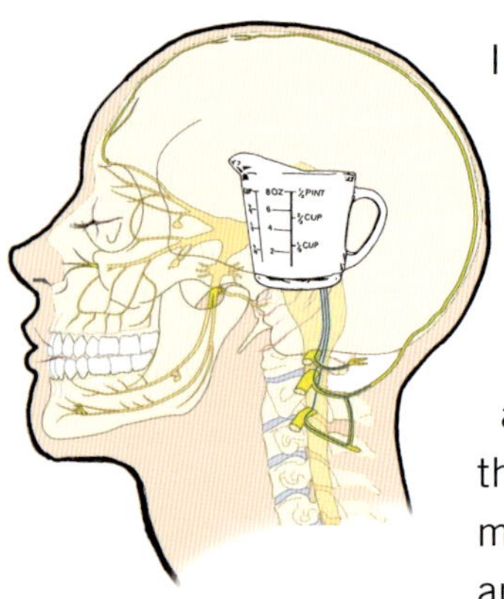

In many ways, headaches work the same way as a measuring cup filling with liquid. At the upper part of the spinal cord is a collection area, similar to a measuring cup. The cup receives and processes information from the upper neck and face joints, muscles, blood vessels and nerves, and then relays it to the brain. The main nerves in the face also send information to the cup for processing.

Additionally, the nervous system relays messages from your environment. All of this information is sent to the measuring cup. As long as the cup doesn't overflow, everything is fine. Once the cup overflows, a headache starts.[5] Emotions and stressors, like failed treatments, family concerns, fear and anxiety, persistent pain, job issues and different explanations for your pain, can also affect how quickly the cup overflows; we'll talk more about that later in the book.

MOST PEOPLE HAVE HEADACHES

Headaches affect many people. It is estimated that at least 80% of all humans experience some form of headache on a regular basis,[6-9] and headaches are among the five most disabling disorders affecting women.[6] Persistent or long-lasting headaches have a severe impact on daily function and life roles. Headaches have a more severe impact than chronic diabetes, high-blood pressure, arthritis and back pain.[10] On a personal level, headaches significantly impact well-being.[11] Persistent headaches decrease productivity, affect relationships with family and friends, cause work related issues with employers, increase anxiety and feelings of helplessness, and lead to anger and frustration.[11] Left untreated, headaches usually increase in frequency from occasional headaches, to more frequent headaches to daily headaches.[12-14]

TYPES OF HEADACHES

Headaches can be caused by many things, including increased stress, tight muscles, bad posture, hormonal changes, allergies, foods, medications, neck injury, indigestion, concussion, high blood pressure and more.[15] Remember the cup? All of this information is sent to the collection area located in the upper part of your spinal cord.

A significant issue that needs to be discussed is the name. Many headache sufferers are aware of names such as migraine, cluster headache, tension headache and neck headache. Does it matter which one you have? The answer for now is "NO." Headache classifications are important only for the people studying and treating headaches.

How you describe your headache allows doctors and physical therapists to determine which structures may be causing the flow into the cup. For example, a sustained neck position could result in tender joints in the neck, limited neck movements and a description of pain in a certain fashion. In this case, the joints could be a significant source in filling the cup. This type of headache receives a specific name, and treatment will be directed toward the joints to lessen the alarm messages filling the cup and ultimately leading to the headache.

In another case, a patient may describe a headache around her menstrual cycle. The pounding and throbbing results in sensitivity to light, dizziness and nausea. This type of headache will be seen as a result of changes in hormones in the blood. Treatment will be directed toward the hormonal issues. All of these strategies will attempt to empty the cup and ease the headache by preventing the flow to the cup. Ultimately, the goal will be to avoid future headaches.

Pain is pain. In medicine, especially in regard to pain, we often overcomplicate issues. Pain is 100% produced by the brain. Pain is produced when the brain perceives there is a threat and protection is needed. All the information described previously from nerves, joints, blood vessels and chemicals is passed from the cup to the brain for interpretation. If there's little threat, pain is not produced. If there's a real threat or the brain perceives a possible threat, pain is produced by the brain. Headache pain can be produced in any part of the head, neck or face.

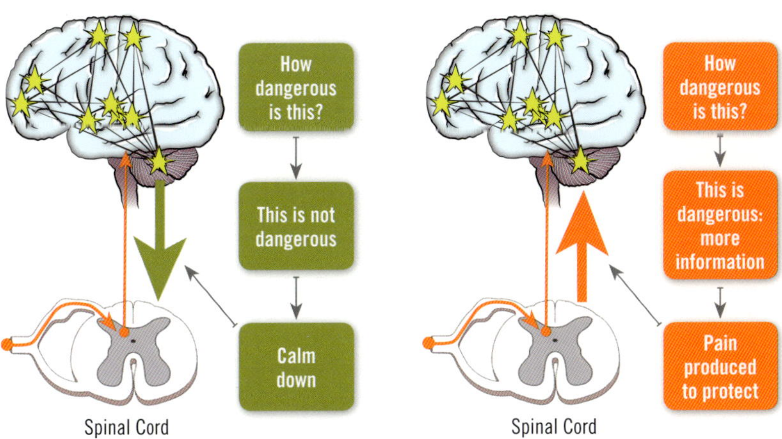

Even though there may be specific causes for headaches, they all share common features in regard to how the pain develops and persists.[5] Neuroscience, the study of nerves and the brain, has increased the understanding of pain and how pain works over the last 10 to 15 years.[1] Additionally, neuroscience research has shown that when people know more about their pain and, more precisely, how their pain works, they experience less pain.[16-18] This book, based on the latest neuroscience, intends to help patients suffering from the pain of a variety of different headaches. This book also intends to help develop a greater understanding of how headache pain works. Last, but certainly not least, this book intends to show you some proven strategies to help ease the pain associated with headaches.

Understanding the Cause

There are many possible headache triggers: reasons for danger messages to be sent to the measuring cup, eventually overflowing into a headache. Sometimes, it only takes messages from one source to overflow the cup. More likely, there are several issues that are all contributing to the overflow.

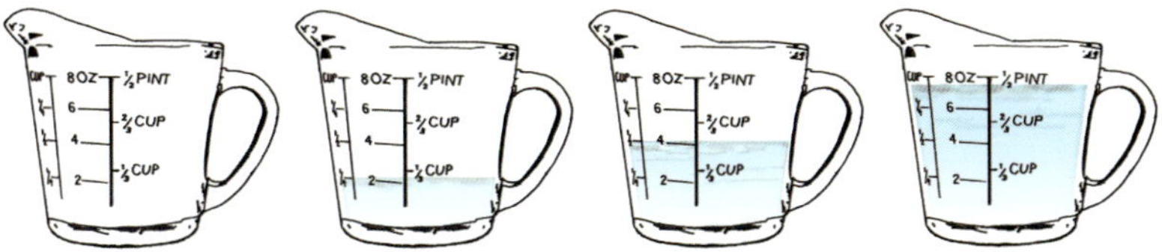

Two common contributors are sensitive tissues and blood vessels in and around the head, neck and face.

3A: Tissues and Blood Vessels

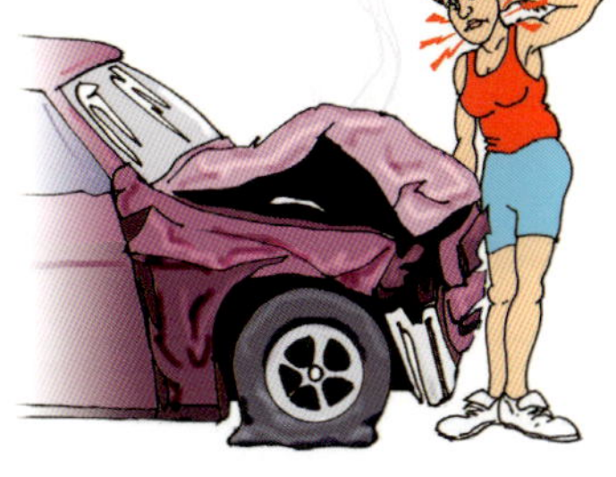

TISSUES: Joints and muscles in the upper neck, head and face are very sensitive and may send a lot of danger messages via the nerves.[19] Remember that these nerves are the alarm system. For example, if a car accident occurs, joints and muscles may be injured, resulting in inflammation and increased spasm. These joints and muscles will send increased danger messages to the relay center to alert you to get some help. Following the car accident, nerves from the face, eyes and head will also send more danger messages. With increasing danger messages being sent to the relay center, the cup begins to fill rapidly and may overflow, causing the brain to produce a headache. The headache pain is normal, expected and protective. In this case, the pain from the headache helps remind you not to move your neck suddenly, as it's just been injured and needs time to recover.

BLOOD VESSELS: There are a large number of blood vessels around the brain.[2] Often, these blood vessels are very sensitive. Because your brain is so important, it makes sense that you have increased security around it. It makes sense as well that the alarm is set at a more sensitive level. Any irritations or changes to the blood vessels, such as pressure, chemicals and hormones, and any changes to the nerves (e.g., stress and anxiety), will result in increased danger messages sent to the collection center, filling the cup. Ultimately, this may lead to headache pain. Think about what happens in a neck injury. The neck muscles tighten up. This causes the local blood vessels to change their blood flow. The cup begins to fill. Danger! Danger! Danger! The local nerves become irritated by the chemicals produced due to the injury. The cup overflows, the brain is alerted and pain is produced to protect you. Treatments directed at the muscles, such as physical therapy stretches and exercises, may loosen up the muscles and increase blood supply. Certain medications may open up some blood flow and even calm the alarm system. The cup is emptied and the headache eases.

WHY DO I HURT WHEN I HAVEN'T HAD AN INJURY?

The previous descriptions showed how injuries may set off the alarm system, overflow the cup and start a headache. Many headache sufferers, however, never experienced an injury. So why do they hurt? Injury and pain are two different issues, as described in the ankle sprain versus bus scenario. With over 300 different types of headaches, there are so many issues, including emotions, stress, foods, genetics and more, that may set off the alarm system. Although it's human to want to know the exact cause of your headache, it may be difficult to narrow it down to one factor. It's likely there are several factors filling the cup and leading to a headache.

Take Away Message:

1. It's great if you can determine a specific trigger for your headache. Addressing this issue can be part of your treatment plan.

2. Don't worry if you can't find a specific trigger. There are many issues that can fill the cup.[20] This means that you need to learn strategies to help ease your headaches, such as the ones that will be discussed in this book.

3. Headaches are a normal form of pain and part of a normal human experience. Everyone gets headaches. The most important issue is to develop a strategy to help yourself during a headache. Better yet, develop strategies to help avoid the headaches.

4. A headache does not necessarily mean something is wrong. It could mean you haven't been sleeping enough or you need to relax a little more, because you're stressed. By making some changes, the cup fills less often and is prevented from overflowing, which can prevent headaches.

Apart from tissues and blood vessels, extra-sensitive nerves play a major role in filling and overflowing the cup: triggering or extending a headache.

3B: Extra-Sensitive Nerves

NERVES: In the example of the rusted nail, you learned that nerves "wake up" and activate the alarm system. When action is taken, the alarm system calms down to its original resting level. In some people, the nerves that "wake up" to alert you to the danger in your tissues calm down very slowly. They remain elevated and "buzzing." In this state, it doesn't take much activity to make the nerves fire off danger messages to the brain — activities like sitting, typing, driving or stressful circumstances, such as an increased work load, a relationship confrontation or a case of indigestion. The nerves become extra sensitive.[19,21,22] In headache patients, their extra-sensitive nervous system causes danger messages to be sent to the cup a lot faster and easier, which fills the cup faster, quickly leading to an overflow and a headache.

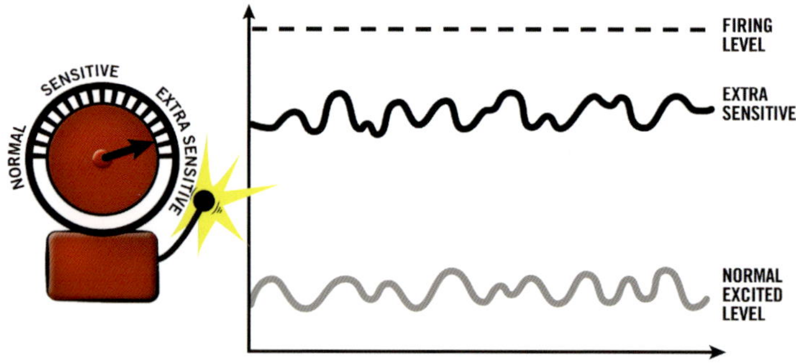

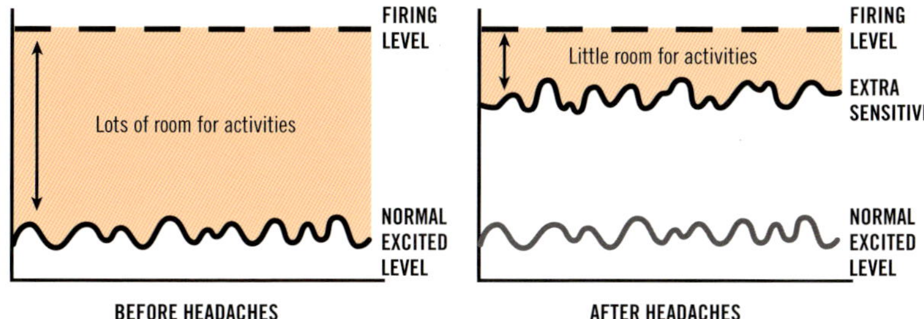

This elevated response is actually normal, but it impedes function and social participation. Look at the two drawings shown above. Before you developed headaches, you were able to perform tasks like driving or working on a computer quite easily and for long periods. In addition, you could experience stressful situations without developing a headache. But since you developed headaches, you've noticed that it only takes a few minutes of the same task or the same amount of daily stress to experience pain. No wonder you think something must be wrong! Think of the activities you used to do, such as exercising, washing loads of laundry, leading a meeting or dealing with daily catastrophes. Now think about how limited you are with the level of pain you're experiencing. The main issue is increased nerve sensitivity.[19,21,22] Your alarm system has become extra sensitive.

ANOTHER WAY TO THINK ABOUT YOUR NERVES IS TO COMPARE THEM TO YOUR HOME ALARM SYSTEM.

Imagine an alarm system is set up in your house. Normal day-to-day activities do not set off the alarm. It's set to be sensitive to bigger issues, such as someone breaking a window. Since you have experienced pain, your alarm system has become so sensitive that when a leaf blows by the house, it sets off the alarm. The alarm system needs to be turned down to decrease its sensitivity.[1]

Check off any answers that fit your situation.

☐ Your activity level before developing a headache has decreased a lot.[11]

☐ You instinctively know you have become more sensitive or even overly sensitive.

☐ You are sensitive to pressure on your skin around your neck, face and head.[25]

☐ When doctors and therapists test you or move your body parts, you are very sensitive.[25]

☐ You are currently on medicine to calm your nerves, such as Cymbalta®, Lyrica® and Neurontin® or anti-depressants, such as Paxil®, Zoloft® and Prozac®.

WHY DID MY NERVES STAY SENSITIVE? THIS DIDN'T HAPPEN TO MY NEIGHBOR.

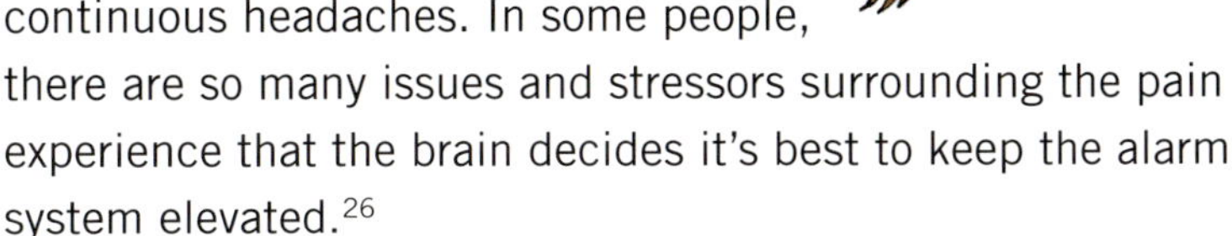

As mentioned before, in some people nerves are slow to calm down. Why is this? Your neighbor, friend or family member had a similar injury, accident or stress in their life; they bounced right back and didn't suffer from continuous headaches. In some people, there are so many issues and stressors surrounding the pain experience that the brain decides it's best to keep the alarm system elevated.[26]

- **Failed treatment:** You may begin to wonder why the treatment isn't working or why the injections helped your neighbor, but not you. You may have attended countless doctors' consultations, therapy visits and more, yet the pain isn't better. In fact, it may even be worse. As long as your brain has questions and concerns, it will keep your alarm system elevated.

- **Family concerns and job issues:** Pain has and will continue to impact your family life and your job. This impact may include concerns about numerous doctor and physical therapy visits, expensive tests, lost work time, frustration and disturbed relationships. In addition, you may have concerns about money, the future or your ability to work. These concerns provide little incentive for your brain to turn down the alarm system.

- **Fear and anxiety:** Considering the failed treatments, various explanations for your pain, job issues and family concerns, there is bound to be a lot of uncertainty. The uncertainty is usually accompanied by some anxiety or fear. This is quite common, but it has been shown that fear of injury, or re-injury, and fear of exercise or movement will keep the alarm system turned on.[27]

- **Persistent pain:** Even though pain is a normal protective mechanism, the pain experience is stressful. Shortly after an injury, accident or stressful time, it's quite normal to experience pain. This pain leads to an elevated alarm system as your brain tries to protect you. Persistent pain is a stressor and can keep the alarm system elevated.

- **Different explanations for your pain:** You may feel more stressed when you're not sure about what is causing your pain and what treatment options you should follow. In addition, you've had different explanations about what to expect. Everyone has an opinion, including family members, friends, doctors and therapists as well as the Internet. All this uncertainty will leave the alarm system elevated as you seek the answers.

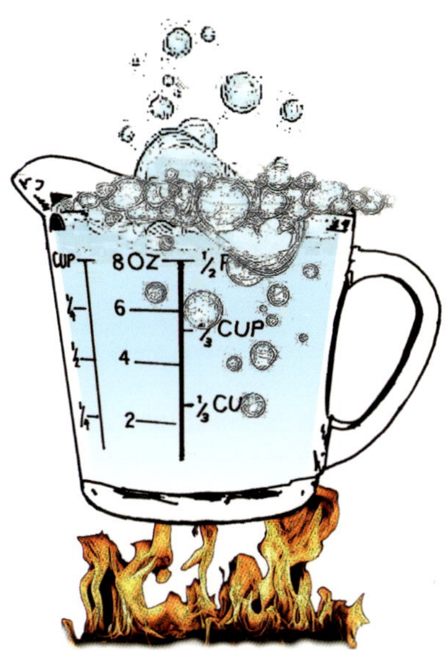

- **Failed Treatment**
- **Fear**
- **Family Concerns**
- **Anxiety**
- **Job Issues**
- **Persistent Pain**
- **Different Explanations**

You can see how many issues are involved in a headache. All the danger messages from your tissues, blood vessels and extra-sensitive nerves are steadily filling the cup, eventually leading to an overflow and a headache. At the same time, your emotions and the stressors surrounding your pain experience work like an open flame, heating the water in the ever-filling cup. This accelerates the cup's overflow — boiling over — causing headache and pain even faster. From this description, it's easy to see how emotions and stressors may lead to headaches. Strategies to deal with these emotions and the stressors need to be developed to turn the flames under the cup down and eventually out. Your headache book will describe various strategies to help with this.

You may have noticed that even beyond the normal sensitivity described, you have become more sensitive to other things, such as cold temperature, bright lights and loud sounds. Inside your nerves, there are various sensors also designed to protect and inform you of any changes in your life.[28,29] Many sensors have been identified, but the following may be of particular interest to you:

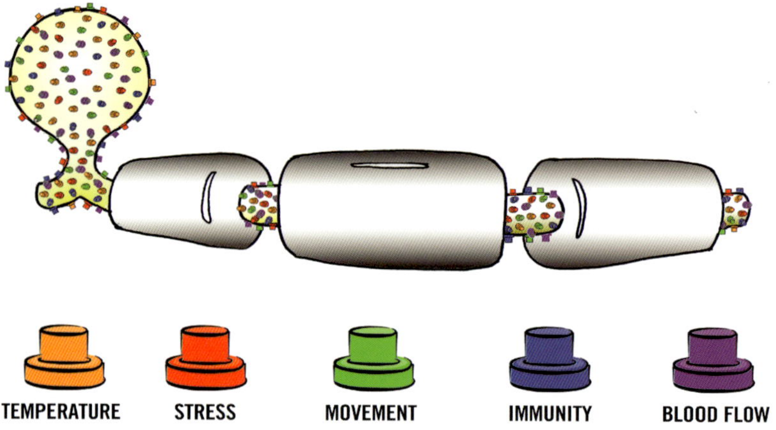

- **Temperature:** There are sensors in nerves that tell you if there is a change in temperature. It is not uncommon to get sensitive to cold temperature and feel more aches and pains in the neck, face and head when it gets cold outside.

- **Stress:** There are sensors in nerves that are sensitive to stress chemicals flowing in your blood. The more stressed, anxious, nervous or upset you are, the more you will experience an increase in aches and pains. The more stress chemicals that run through your body, the more stress sensors are activated.

- **Blood flow and pressure:** There are sensors in your nerves that are sensitive to the amount of blood around your tissues. When blood flow slows down slightly, after working on the computer too long, for example, these sensors "wake up" and make the nerves sensitive.

- **Movement and pressure:** There are sensors in your nerves that are sensitive to movement. For example, strenuous arm exercises or carrying heavy bags may activate a few more sensors and make the nerves extra sensitive for a little while.

- **Immunity:** When you are sick with the flu, for example, there are many immune molecules floating through your body, helping you deal with the illness. This also happens following injury or a stressful event. Recent research shows that when you are really worried about an injured or painful body part, or an underlying cause of your headache, you'll have an immune response. Nerves have sensors telling them of the increased immune molecules, and the immune chemicals produced can make you ache.

KEY POINTS ABOUT NERVE SENSORS:

✓ To date we have discovered hundreds of different sensors.

✓ There are sensors sensitive to light.

✓ There are sensors sensitive to various hormones in your blood.

✓ There are sensors sensitive to the blood flowing through your body.

✓ There are sensors sensitive to various chemical compounds.

✓ When you develop headaches, your nerves increase their sensitivity to protect you. This is a normal response that happens in every human being.

✓ These sensors are constantly updated based on your environment.

We now know that changes in hormones, blood pressure, light, sound, touch, illness, stress, anxiety, allergies and more are all capable of setting off the alarm system, activating danger messages and filling the cup. As a result of these changes, you can develop headaches. The good news is that these sensors change every few days and can be influenced by the treatments described in your headache book.

3C: Processing Danger Messages

The brain's processing of danger messages from the tissues and environment is important in understanding your headache. For years, it was generally believed that there was a single pain area in the brain. When you sprain your ankle, the light bulb flashes on and there it is. Pain! If pain were so simple, it would be easy to cut this area out of the brain and all pain would be gone. When you have a pain experience, such as a headache, it is now well established by scientists that various areas of your brain are involved in processing this pain experience.[30,31] These areas then connect and form a pain map. This happens for any and all kinds of pain, including headaches. Patients diagnosed with low back pain, neck pain, fibromyalgia, chronic headaches and chronic fatigue syndrome have very similar brain areas that light up during a pain experience. Another way to think of it is an airline map. If you page through any airline magazine, you will notice the map showing where the airline flies. With all the areas in your brain processing danger messages from the relay center, you have developed something similar to an airline map in the brain. In addition, it's important for you to know that, just as in real life, people fly different airlines. Each person that experiences pain uses similar areas of the brain, but the pathways are different. Pain is individualized, which makes it so hard to treat. You need treatment tailored to your pain. Your headache is unique to you.

These areas that light up in a pain experience also deal with other tasks. If your headache pain uses these areas, they may struggle to perform their best, leading to further frustration and suffering. The most common areas used in pain are as follows:

- **Sensation:** Each body part, such as your upper back, neck, shoulder or face, is represented in the brain, in essence forming a map of your body so you can recognize body parts. Your brain tells you where you are experiencing sensations in your body, including pain. If pain uses this area, you may experience pain that spreads into the neck and upper back. This is normal and helps therapists realize just how much the headache is impacting your function.

- **Movement:** The areas that plan, coordinate and execute your movements are also busy protecting you. Maybe some muscles needed to protect you will stiffen up and not allow you to turn your neck as far as before or move your shoulders as before.

- **Focus and concentration:** The areas dealing with focus and concentration are also busy dealing with your pain experience. People in pain often describe feeling as if they're in a fog when they are in pain, which means the area that deals with focus is busy helping out with pain.

- **Fear:** The emotional areas of the brain dealing with fear, such as fear of pain or even fear of activity increasing the pain are called upon, especially when pain is poorly understood. Fears, anxieties and emotions may be increased during your headache.

- **Memory:** The areas of the brain dealing with memory are busy. They remember previous similar experiences and call on those strategies to help. People in pain may experience some issues with memory. This is expected and easily explained.

- **Motivation:** The area dealing with motivation is now used to process pain instead of motivating.

- **Stress responses:** There are specialized areas in the brain that deal with stress. These centers control the release of various stress chemicals, such as adrenaline and cortisol, into the body to help protect you. These centers also control sleep, appetite, body weight and body temperature.

KEY ISSUE:

The key issue here is that many brain areas are involved in all pain experiences, including your headache. These areas communicate with each other to discuss the appropriate action. This communication influences the brain's normal tasks. Other common functions, such as memory, sleep and focus, become neglected. This can easily be explained, is not a big deal and is part of dealing with the pain.

A common, but unfortunate, saying is that "pain is in your head." The saying implies that it's not real; it's fabricated and it's only in your mind. This is not true. Yes, pain is located in your head, within your brain. When you have pain, the brain is very active processing it. How your brain processes information determines the pain you experience. So, yes, your pain experience is in your head, but it is very real. It can be measured, and it can be changed for the better.

Understanding What Will Help

In Sections 1-3, the development of a headache was described as filling a measuring cup, which results in a headache if it overflows. Additionally, we described how emotions and stress work like an open flame heating the cup, which can increase the chance of the cup boiling over. To treat headaches, we can do the following:

STOP FILLING THE CUP, or EMPTY THE CUP.

Many people with repeated episodes of headache have several issues that fill their cup. After thorough examination, these issues can be identified and treatment can be designed to stop input to the cup or possibly even empty it. This can vary from treatment of the neck joints and muscles, to hormonal balance, to a change in diet, to drinking enough water, to taking care of high blood pressure and so forth.

EXTINGUISH THE FIRE UNDER THE CUP.

Many people experience stress in their lives. Life is filled with many worries, especially when people are in pain. These include uncertainties about pain and struggles coping with pain. Finding ways to deal with the stress and emotions

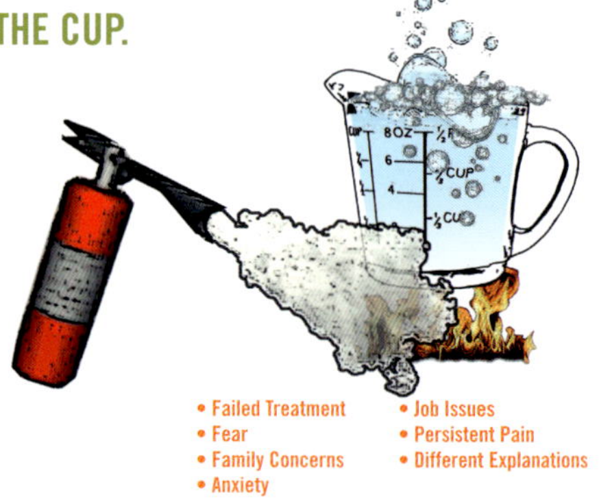

due to your pain can, in essence, extinguish the fire under the cup, which will also ease your headaches.

Certainly, headaches are complex; however, all the current treatments directed at treating various forms of headaches work on the principles outlined in this book. Depending on the issues that may be filling and overflowing your cup and fueling the fire, there are a variety of possible treatments.

1. Knowledge

Education is therapy. Gaining an understanding of the neuroscience of your headache pain will undoubtedly ease some fears, explain some unknowns and provide some hope. This alone will move you toward recovery.[18,32] How you think and process pain are directly linked to how much pain you experience, and a major cause of your pain is an extra-sensitive nervous system. If you understand those two concepts, you are well on your way to recovery. In fact, studies have shown that once you understand what is causing your pain, your nerves immediately begin to calm.

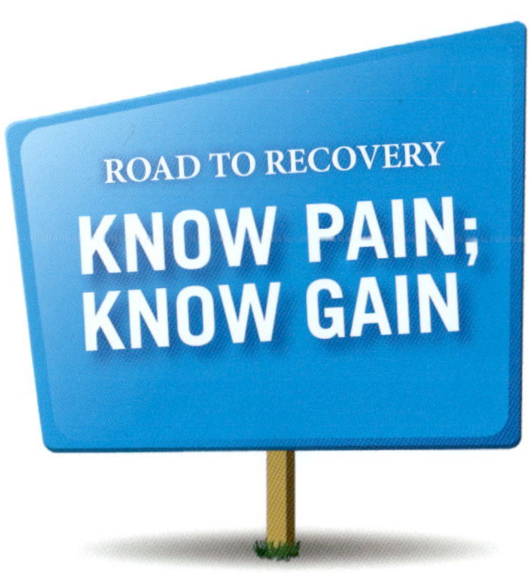

The images below show the brain scan of a patient with years of pain. In the first row, the patient is resting and there is little brain activity. Remember the pain map or airline map in the head? In the next row of scans, the patient does a painful task, and the brain is very active dealing with pain. Notice all the red blobs in the scan. The third row of scans shows the patient's brain doing the same painful task as during the second scan. The difference is because the patient has just completed a 30-minute neuroscience education session that covered similar material found in your headache book. You will notice a significant reduction in the brain's activity, which is a way to show pain has eased.

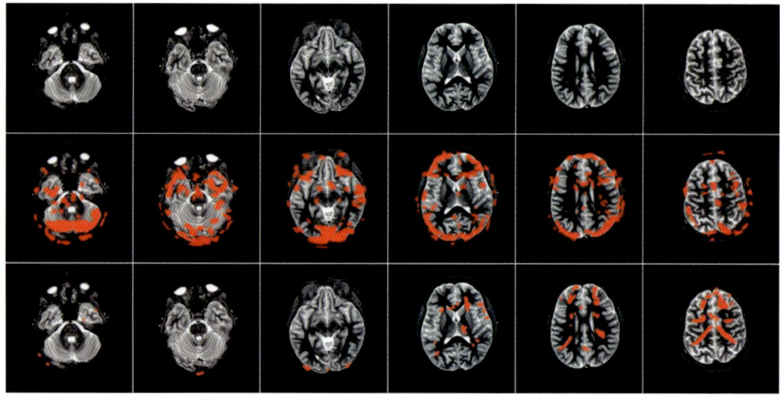

It may seem too simple, but education really is therapy. The good news is this: since you're now half-way finished reading this book, the same process has already started. Additionally, this newly gained knowledge of your pain, such as learning about sensitive nerves and how your brain is very busy dealing with pain, will have a calming effect on your extra-sensitive nerves. Remember, this is a sophisticated alarm system, and if you've been struggling with headache pain for a prolonged period, the system will turn down a little bit at a time.[19,21,22]

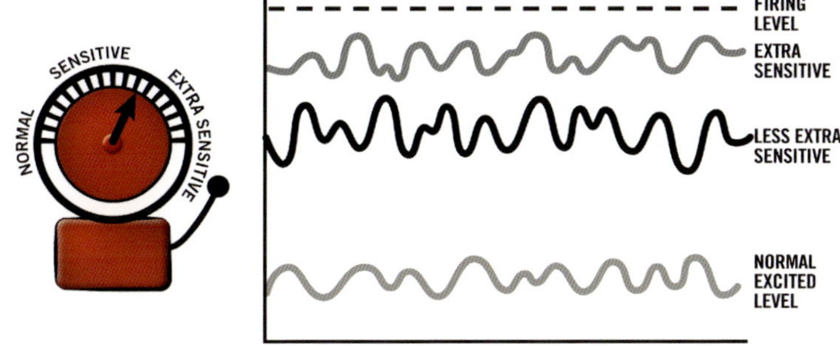

Develop a saying or mantra to explain your pain to yourself and anyone interested in your pain. By rehearsing it and saying it over and over, the brain's belief as well as the brain's activity will be strongly influenced. This includes taking away uncertainty, which typically fuels pain. Below are examples you can use or adapt. Better yet, make your own.

- *Hurt does not equal harm.*

- *My headache pain does not mean something is wrong. My nerves are just extra sensitive. There are many things I can do to calm down the extra-sensitive nerves and ease my headache.*

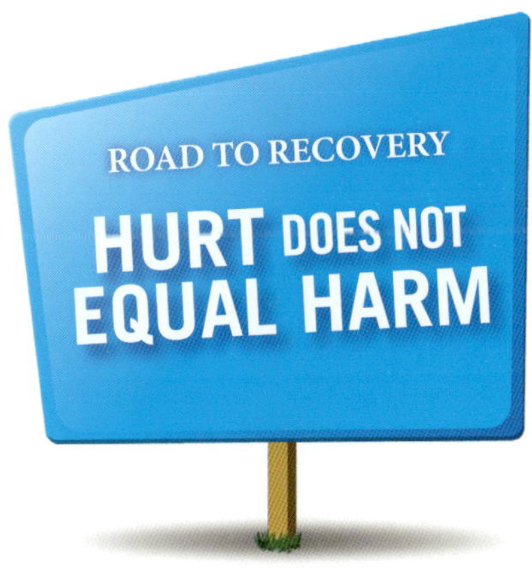

2. Manual Therapy

In Section 2, we described how the joints, muscles and nerves of the upper part of the neck have a direct feed to your headache cup.[5] When these tissues become stiff, a little

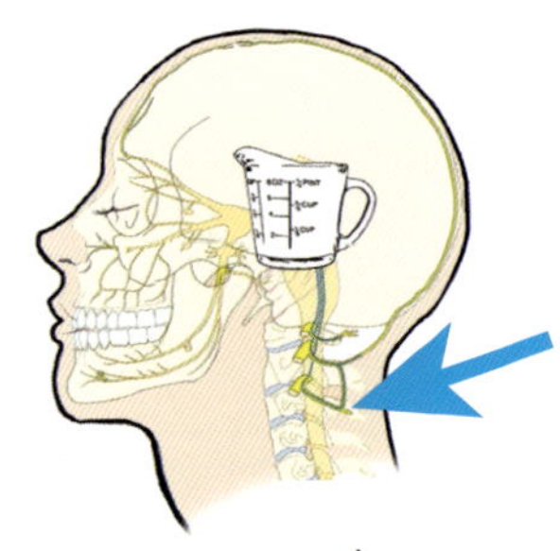

swollen or sensitive, they send more danger messages to the cup. Additionally, if the joints and muscles get a little stiff and restricted, they increase the alarm system messages, restrict much-needed blood flow to the nerves, and change some of the local chemicals. This may in turn cause the alarm system to fire off more danger messages. Simply stated—if the joints and muscles of the upper neck move more freely, the alarm system will calm down a little and more blood and oxygen will be available for the nerves. This will help ease a headache by not filling the cup too much. Manual therapy is a strategy that has shown a lot of benefit in helping these tissues move better.[33,34] Manual therapy is passive movement techniques applied to the neck by a physical therapist aiming to optimize the movement of your tissues.[35] Yes, active exercises can also help; you'll read about these later. As a means to have specific joints move, manual therapy can direct treatment to specific levels. You could view these treatments as a jumpstart to get tissues to loosen up. Manual therapy followed by active home exercises is what you need to do to help keep the upper neck moving.

3. Specific Neck Exercises

In line with manual therapy, exercise
may also help loosen up the joints
and muscles of the upper neck.[34]
Since muscles span large areas, for
example, some muscles you touch at the
back of your neck cover the upper back as well,
exercise should focus on all the muscles around
the upper back and neck. Free, comfortable movement
of the neck allows blood and oxygen to flow in and around
the neck, head and face, reducing the feed into the headache
cup. An added benefit of exercise is the fact that you can
help yourself. By learning a few simple, easy stretches and
range-of-motion exercises, you can help ease your headache
pain or even help prevent the onset of a headache. Take
regular breaks at a computer station by doing a few stretches
and neck movements; it may work wonders as you take control
of your headache.

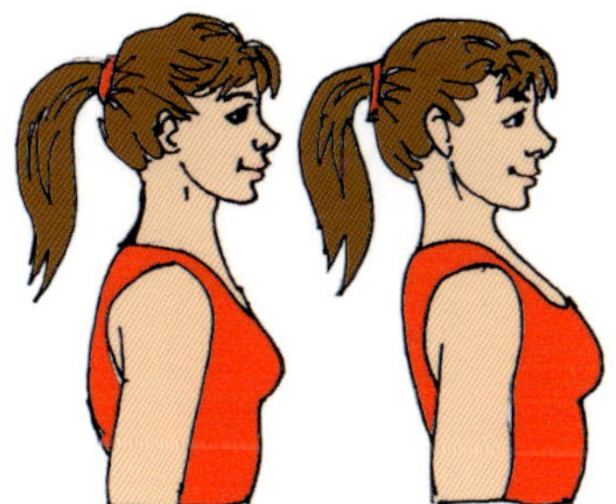
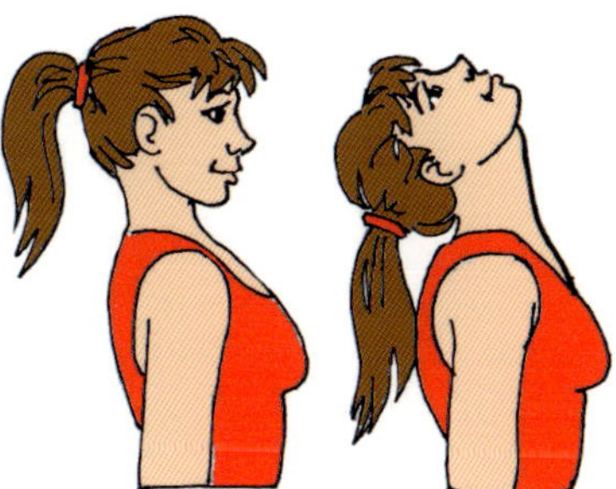

4. Aerobic Exercises

Research has shown that aerobic exercise, which gets your heart pumping a little faster and pumps blood and oxygen through your body, helps to calm nerves down.[36,37] Don't worry; there is no need to run marathons or climb mountains. Studies have shown that brisk walking — between 10-20 minutes — is all that is needed to have a calming effect on nerves. In fact, most people can easily get there just by raising their heart rate 20 beats a minute.[38] Also, remember that if you pump blood and oxygen through your body regularly, you will achieve the following benefits:

✓ Decreased headaches and pain

✓ Decreased muscle soreness and fatigue

✓ Improved sleep

✓ Improved enjoyment of the taste of food

✓ Increased weight loss

✓ Decreased stress levels

✓ Decreased mood swings

✓ Decreased or loss of depression

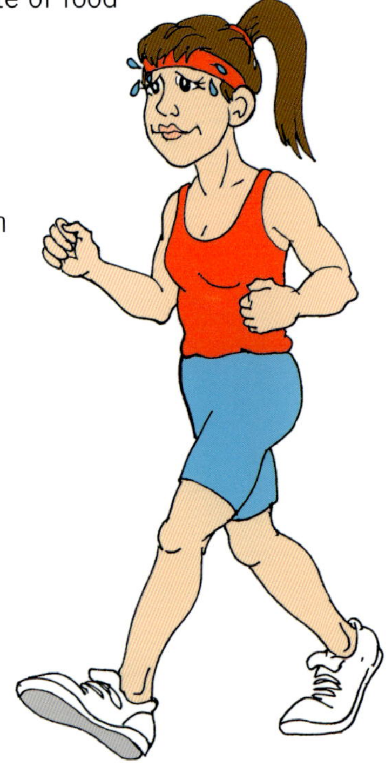

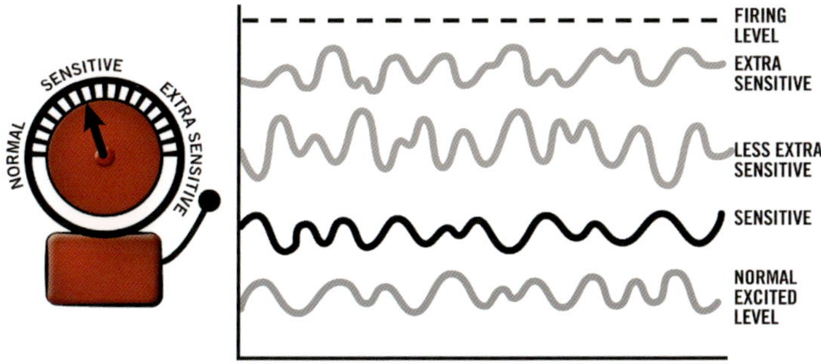

HELPFUL EXERCISE STRATEGIES[1]

There are many strategies you can try to help you exercise and calm down. In fact, books have been written about just that. Here are some helpful strategies people have used over the years.

- **Start small:** Start with three to four minutes of exercise. Every two days, add a minute until you reach 15-20 minutes of regular exercise. Walking is an easy option. You can substitute walking with biking or swimming. Remember that increasing your heart rate is the main goal.

- **Make a plan:** On paper, write down a plan that includes where, when and how long you will exercise.

- **Take rests:** Don't exercise every day. Schedule days off. Exercise five days a week.

- **Get a partner:** Exercise with a friend, neighbor or family member. Explain your plan so they can help.

- **Back off:** Many people in pain are doing too much exercise. Pace yourself.

- **Get away:** Avoid working out at home. Get outside in the fresh air. If it's cold, walk in the mall. Home is usually filled with stressful issues, such as housework and family needs.

- **Log your progress:** Start a log book or journal. After each workout, write what you did. Record some positive thoughts about your workout, your day and your progress.

- **Set a goal:** Be specific. It may be to complete a loop around the park or to participate in a charity walk by a certain date. Plan and prepare.

- **Breathe deeply:** When you exercise, remember to breathe. Take nice big breaths. The mixture of blood and oxygen flushing through your body will help calm your nerves and excite your brain.

5. Medication

First, all questions about your medication should be directed to your doctor. With all your medical experiences, you are probably aware that pharmaceutical companies have developed a series of drugs to calm nerves. Skillful delivery of medication may be helpful for some patients. Patients affected with severe headaches can be especially helped by medication.

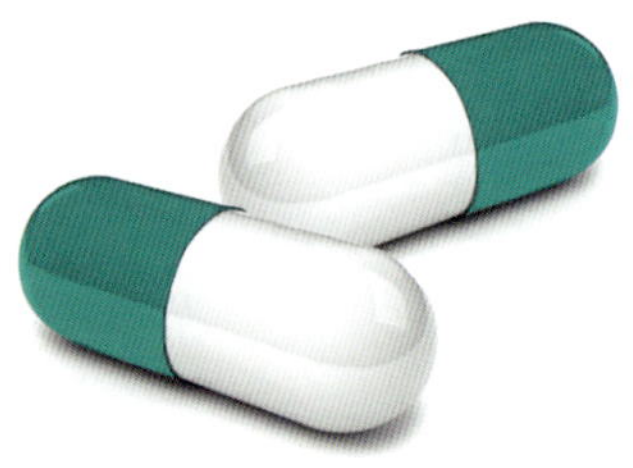

Did you know the brain produces the most potent pain medicine on the planet, helping people survive severe injuries while experiencing little or no pain?[39] The brain produces these "happy chemicals" that then have a calming effect and change the danger messages. This scenario is described as a "wet brain." It's juicy and full of good, healthy medicine, which can be released to help you when you're in pain from stubbing a toe or dealing with a bad headache. People with persistent pain have "dry brains." The medicine has dried up to make you more sensitive to protect yourself.[19,21,22]

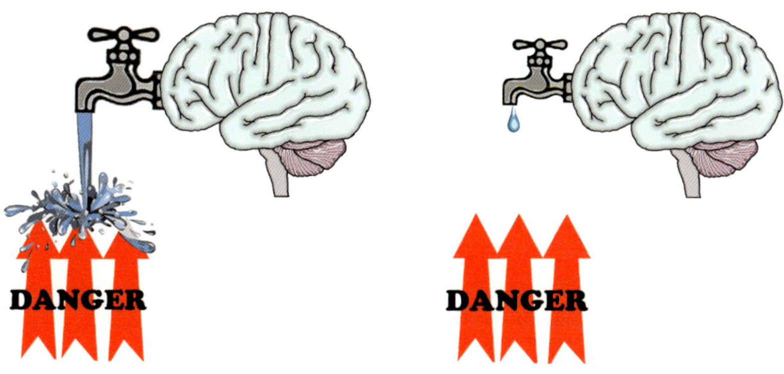

Unfortunately, people who have struggled with pain for a long time have this drug cabinet affected in a negative way. As the brain becomes more worried and interested in what's going on with your headache, it takes the numbing medicine out of the body, making you more sensitive to get you to protect yourself. This is one reason why you have developed some increased sensitivity to movement, light, sounds, stress and so forth. When experiencing persistent headache pain, your brain produces less of the medicine that helps you deal with pain on a daily basis. Is this permanent? No. It can it be changed in the following ways:

- **Knowledge:** Increasing knowledge of how your pain works, such as reading this book, allows for greater understanding and less fear and anxiety.[40] With less fear and anxiety, and a greater realistic understanding of your headache pain experience, the brain will once again produce increased numbing medicine to help.

- **Aerobic exercise:** After approximately 10 minutes of moderate aerobic exercise, the brain produces more of a calming effect on nerves. Pumping blood and oxygen around nerves also calms them down.[37,38]

- **Medication:** Low-dose anti-depressants are able to gently open this medicine cabinet in the brain.[36]

- **Food:** Various foods may help decrease pain by increasing some of the "happy chemicals" in the brain and spinal cord. For example, some carbohydrates produce a calming effect, since carbohydrates contain tryptophan, which is turned into calming medicine in the brain.[41]

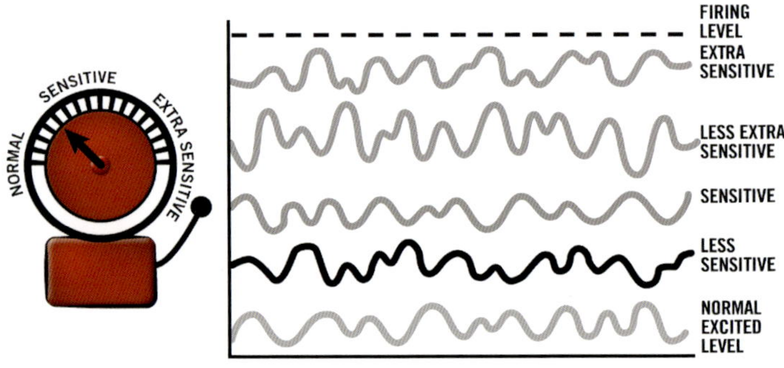

6. Cooling Nerves Down

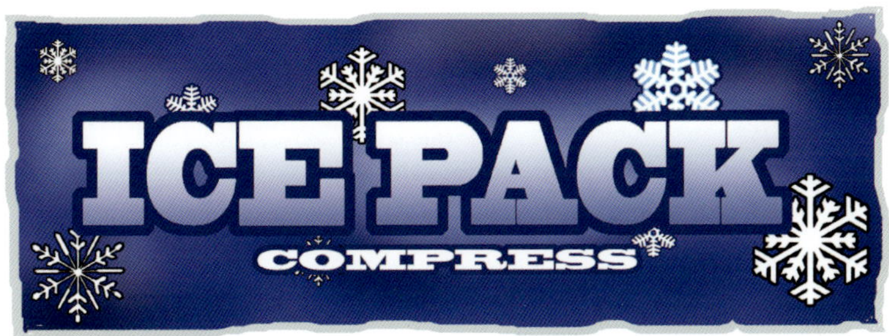

The main theme of the book is the increasing danger messages sent to the cup by your extra-sensitive alarm system. It is now well established that danger messages actually slow down when a body part is cooled with ice.[42] This is especially true for the extra-sensitive nerves in the upper part of your neck. Take three or four minutes to ice the neck and calm the nerves down a little. Want some more good news? Ice also increases blood flow in tissues, which is very important in headaches. The cooling effect will get blood vessels to narrow a little. After they are cool, they'll open up again, flushing extra blood and oxygen around the sensitive nerves and helping ease the pain.

7. Breathing and Relaxation

By now you should realize that pumping more blood and oxygen around nerves helps calm them down. This calming effect decreases the danger messages sent to the cup, making it less full, thus treating or avoiding a headache. In addition to relaxation, another important strategy is implementing breathing exercises. Deep, slow, relaxed breathing will help. Muscles can better relax, and you will calm down. Deeper, relaxed breathing should form part of a healthy routine of exercising, relaxing and gaining more knowledge about your headache pain. One last thought: Think about how nice it feels to take a relaxing, deep sigh of relief after some good news.

There are obviously many techniques and philosophies regarding relaxation. The message here is simply to make time for you. Turn the lights down, turn the television off and do some relaxing, resting and breathing.

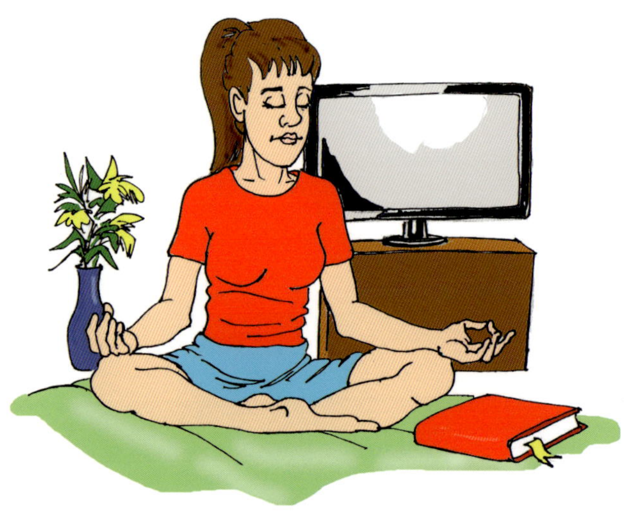

8. Sleep

This is a huge topic and a very important one, as well. Numerous sleep studies on pain, including headache pain, have revealed a lack of deep, restorative sleep as a contributing factor.[43] Few things have as big an effect on our health as sleep. At least eight hours of sleep is needed for most people. Americans average six hours a night, and people in pain average less. Even if you sleep a lot, you never feel refreshed when you wake. Sleep deprivation has been linked to increased rates of pain, obesity, depression and other health-related disorders. Changing sleep habits is hard, but important for your recovery. There are many helpful sleep strategies, including the following:

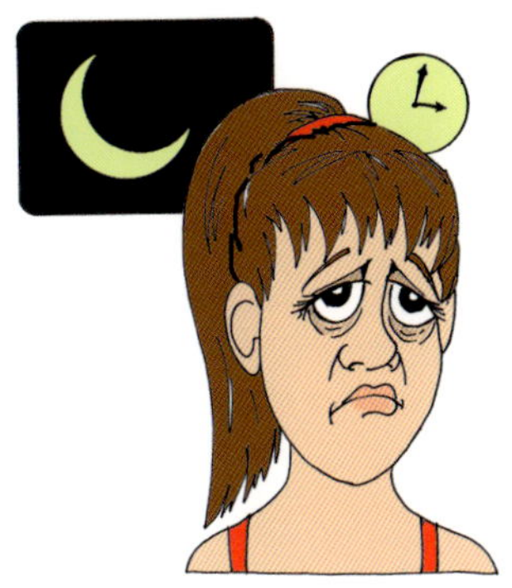

- **Shut off:** Shut the lights, television and computer off because they stimulate your nervous system and brain.

- **Set time:** Have a set time to go to bed. It has been shown the more time you sleep before midnight, the more refreshed you are in the morning.

- **Naps:** If you sleep during the day for more than a 20 minute nap, it will have a negative effect on your much needed night sleep. If you need a nap or two, make them power naps of 20 minutes of less.

- **Caffeine:** No caffeine late in the afternoon or evening.

- **Notes:** Park your ideas. When you have a lot of stuff running through your head, write it down so the brain can go to sleep.

- **Dark and cool:** Darken and cool your bedroom.

- **Bed buddies:** No kids or animals in your bed.

- **Alcohol:** Limit alcohol in the evening to avoid bathroom breaks in the middle of the night when you need the deep, resting phases of sleep.

- **Water:** Limit water intake in the evening to avoid bathroom breaks.

- **Close your eyes:** If you find it hard to fall asleep, close your eyes and force yourself to sleep. Similarly, if you are wide awake in the morning before it's your time to wake, keep your eyes closed and rest. After doing this for a few days, these closed-eye sessions will transfer into sleep.

- **Exercise:** You sleep better when you exercise regularly

9. Consider How You Sit

It is important, once again, to realize headaches are usually not due to one single issue; there are usually several issues feeding into the cup. An issue that is often talked about in headache patients is posture, especially sitting posture. By now, based on everything you know about headaches from this book, you have become a headache master. You likely realize that prolonged sitting in a bad posture will add stress to your muscles, causing them to tighten up, joints to load too much, blood flow to decrease and the alarm system to wake up more and more, eventually leading to a headache. Correcting your sitting posture or the way you carry your upper body can have a big influence on decreasing the danger messages. Below are some helpful sitting tips.

- Limit the amount of time you sit in one position. Take frequent breaks. This will allow you to get out of these positions. Furthermore, if you get away from your desk, you will be able to get some extra blood flowing around your extra-sensitive nerves. Go get a drink of water, which will keep you hydrated; your heart rate will increase a little and get some blood flowing. This will give your tired muscles and joints a little break.

- Put a rolled towel, pillow or lumbar support behind your back to help you keep an upright posture.

- When working on a computer, put the monitor at a level that keeps you in an upright posture.

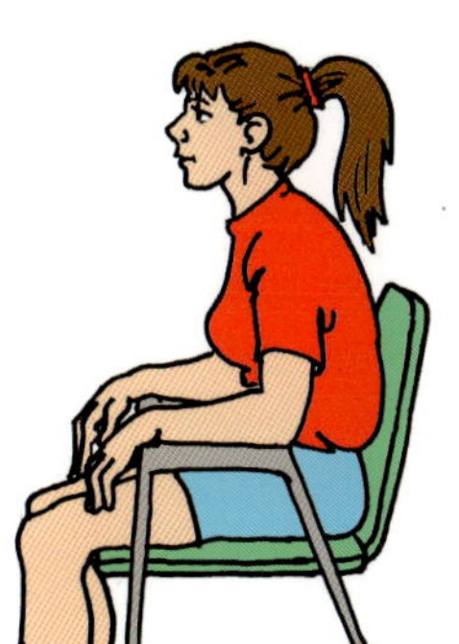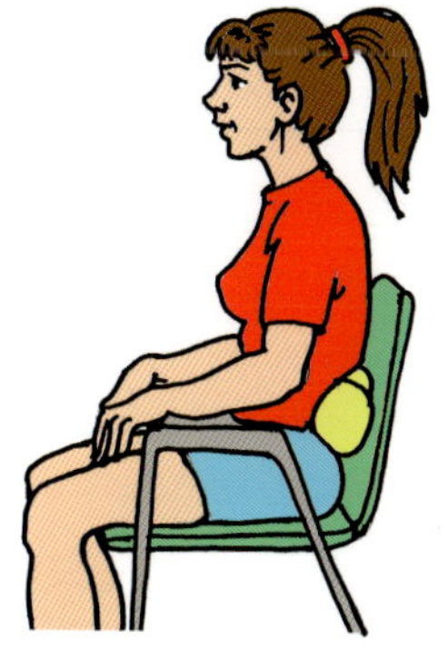

10. Stress Management

By now you should realize that many of the strategies we have
described are part of an overall life coping strategy. Yes, you
have a headache and it's likely impacted your life. Take your
life back. Use this book. Read it again and again. Become an
expert on your headache. Remember, you own your headache.
Then, make some much needed changes in your life, such
as exercise, rest, relaxation, sleep and more. Make time for
yourself. We often find people in pain have little or no time for
themselves. Set some goals. Restart an old hobby. Make time.

Part of managing your stress is knowing how to deal with a
bad day. Having a bad day and being worried about what to
do when a headache comes, presents incredible stress. These
stresses will boil the cup over and start a headache, making an
already bad day worse. On a bad day, consider the following:

- **Realize it's normal:** If you suffer from headaches, there
  is a chance you will have a headache again. The treatments
  in this book are backed by good research and years of
  treating headache patients. This information can and will
  help you. The reality is that you will still have headaches,
  but they should become less frequent and less severe
  over time. When a headache happens, calm down and tell
  yourself, *"It's OK; I expected it. It's normal. Now, let's do
  something about it."*

- **Problem solve:** If possible, try to
  identify the trigger issues for your
  headache. By identifying them, you
  can develop strategies to deal with
  similar situations in the future.
  Remember stress and emotions
  can also trigger headaches.

- **Reduce pain:** Use any measure possible to ease pain. You may have found a little heat or cold to help. Perhaps a certain medicine eases the pain. The faster you can decrease the actual pain experience, the better off you will be. Know what your strategy is and have it ready.

- **Move:** Once you stop, think and take action to ease some pain, start moving as soon as you can. This includes your simple, easy-to-perform neck exercises as well as a little walking. Don't feel inclined to do all your stretches, or your typical distance, but do some. Blood flow and oxygen is essential for recovery.

- **Get away:** If you are in the midst of a stressful scenario or environment, get away. At a job or at your desk, stand up and walk to the drinking fountain or rest room while taking some nice deep breaths. Better yet, skip the closest one and head for one further down the hall to get a few more cleansing breaths and steps. If at home with kids and noise, step outside the house; maybe walk a little down the road, turn around and come back.

- **No on/off switch:** On a bad day, do not draw a line through your list of things you must do and go lay down on the couch, or cancel all work activities and go home. These are very passive ways to deal with your pain and are not very helpful. Instead, keep a few tasks on your list, reschedule a few for tomorrow and still get some work done. For example, the housewife can decide to at least do one load of laundry and sweep one floor as opposed to all the laundry and all the floors. The business person can reschedule a few meetings and tasks for tomorrow, but complete other tasks today.

A final part of the overall stress management is pacing. Find an easy, flowing rhythm to your day that's in line with the coping strategies listed. Plan your days. Pace yourself. Make time for yourself. A day that gets 75% of your tasks completed without a headache beats a day where 100% of your tasks are completed, but the result is a three-day headache.

Your Headache Book Is Finished, But It's Time To Get Started

When you've been suffering from headache pain for as long as you have, it's not uncommon to want someone to just make the pain go away. The information presented here is based on hundreds of research studies and thousands of personal stories. Regardless of the best medicine, education session or personal coaching, the decision is ultimately yours. It's easy to read a little book on pain, but now it's time to get started. You need to apply what you've learned about your body's alarm system and your headaches to your life. Remember that the alarm system is very sophisticated, and it's been set on high for a long time. You can't expect the system to go from high to low over night. As you begin to apply the strategies in this book to your life, you'll begin to reclaim your life and your pain will begin to diminish. It will continue to diminish steadily over time. Remember that pain is a normal part of life, but living in pain is not.

Scientific Support for Your Recovery

1. Louw A, Puentedura EJ. *Therapeutic Neuroscience Education*. Vol 1. Minneapolis, MN: OPTP; 2013.
2. Carter R. *The Human Brain Book*. First ed. New York: Dorling Kindersley Limited; 2009.
3. Louw A, Butler DS, Diener I, Puentedura EJ. Development of a preoperative neuroscience educational program for patients with lumbar radiculopathy. *American journal of physical medicine & rehabilitation/Association of Academic Physiatrists*. May 2013;92(5):446-452.
4. Moseley GL. A pain neuromatrix approach to patients with chronic pain. *Man Ther*. Aug 2003;8(3):130-140.
5. Louw A, Mintken P, Puentedura L. Neuophysiologic Effects of Neural Mobilization Maneuvers. In: Fernandez-De Las Penas C, Arendt-Nielsen L, Gerwin RD, eds. *Tension-type and Cervicogenic Headache*. Boston: Jones and Bartlett; 2009:231-245.
6. Stovner L, Hagen K, Jensen R, et al. The global burden of headache: a documentation of headache prevalence and disability worldwide. *Cephalalgia*. Mar 2007;27(3):193-210.
7. Jensen R, Stovner LJ. Epidemiology and comorbidity of headache. *Lancet Neurol*. Apr 2008;7(4):354-361.
8. Pfaffenrath V, Kaube H. Diagnostics of cervicogenic headache. *Funct Neurol*. Apr-Jun 1990;5(2):159-164.
9. Jensen R. Diagnosis, epidemiology, and impact of tension-type headache. *Curr Pain Headache Rep*. Dec 2003;7(6):455-459.
10. Solomon S. Diagnosis of primary headache disorders. Validity of the International Headache Society criteria in clinical practice. *Neurol Clin*. Feb 1997;15(1):15-26.
11. Diener JH. The impact of cervicogenic headache on patients attending a private physiotherapy practice in Cape Town. *South African Journal of Physiotherapy*. 2001;57(1).
12. Dodick DW, Capobianco DJ. Treatment and management of cluster headache. *Curr Pain Headache Rep*. Feb 2001;5(1):83-91.
13. Spierings EL, Ranke AH, Schroevers M, Honkoop PC. Chronic daily headache: a time perspective. *Headache*. Apr 2000;40(4):306-310.
14. Silberstein SD, Lipton RB. Headache epidemiology. Emphasis on migraine. *Neurol Clin*. May 1996;14(2):421-434.
15. Darof RB. Classification and diagnostic criteria for headache disorders, cranial neuralgias and facial pain. *Cephalagia*. 1988;8 (Suppl 7):1-96.
16. Louw A, Diener I, Butler DS, Puentedura EJ. The effect of neuroscience education on pain, disability, anxiety, and stress in chronic musculoskeletal pain. *Archives of physical medicine and rehabilitation*. Dec 2011;92(12):2041-2056.
17. Moseley GL, Hodges PW, Nicholas MK. A randomized controlled trial of intensive neurophysiology education in chronic low back pain. *Clinical Journal of Pain*. 2004;20:324-330.
18. Moseley L. Combined physiotherapy and education is efficacious for chronic low back pain. *Aust J Physiother*. 2002;48(4):297-302.
19. Louw A. *Whiplash: An Alarming Message from your Nerves*. Minneapolis: OPTP; 2012.
20. Maizels M. Understanding the headache patient with complex comorbidities: a primary care physician's perspective. *Headache*. Oct 2006;46 Suppl 3: S160-162.

21. Louw A. *Your Nerves Are Having Back Surgery.* Minneapolis: OPTP; 2012.
22. Louw A. *Why Do I Hurt? A Neuroscience Approach to Pain.* Minneapolis: OPTP; 2013.
23. Louw A, Puentedura EL, Mintken P. Use of an abbreviated neuroscience education approach in the treatment of chronic low back pain: A case report. *Physiotherapy theory and practice.* Jul 3 2011.
24. Smart KM, Blake C, Staines A, Doody C. Self-reported pain severity, quality of life, disability, anxiety and depression in patients classified with 'nociceptive', 'peripheral neuropathic' and 'central sensitisation' pain. The discriminant validity of mechanisms-based classifications of low back (+/-leg) pain. *Manual therapy.* Apr 2012;17(2):119-125.
25. Drummond PD, Knudsen L. Central pain modulation and scalp tenderness in frequent episodic tension-type headache. *Headache.* Mar 2011;51(3):375-383.
26. Kendall NAS, Linton SJ, Main CJ. *Guide to assessing psychosocial yellow flags in acute low back pain: risk factors for long term disability and work loss.* Wellington: Accident Rehabilitation & Compensation Insurance Corporation of New Zealand and the National Health Committee; 1997.
27. Waddell G, Newton M, Henderson I, al. e. A fear-avoidance beliefs questionnaire (FABQ) and the role of fear avoidance beliefs in chronic low back pain and disability. *Pain.* 1993;52:157-168.
28. Devor M. Sodium channels and mechanisms of neuropathic pain. *J Pain.* Jan 2006;7(1 Suppl 1):S3-S12.
29. Devor M. The pathophysiology and anatomy of damaged nerve. In: Wall PD, Melzack R, eds. *Textbook of Pain.* Edinburgh: Churchill Livingstone; 1984:49-64.
30. Puentedura EJ, Louw A. A neuroscience approach to managing athletes with low back pain. *Phys Ther Sport.* Aug 2012;13(3):123-133.
31. Flor H. The image of pain. Paper presented at: Annual scientific meeting of The Pain Society (Britain)2003; Glasgow, Scotland.
32. Moseley GL. Widespread brain activity during an abdominal task markedly reduced after pain physiology education: fMRI evaluation of a single patient with chronic low back pain. *Aust J Physiother.* 2005;51(1):49-52.
33. Jull G, Trott P, Potter H, et al. A randomized controlled trial of exercise and manipulative therapy for cervicogenic headache. *Spine.* Sep 1 2002;27(17):1835-1843; discussion 1843.
34. Fernandez-de-Las-Penas C. Physical therapy and exercise in headache. *Cephalalgia.* Jul 2008;28 Suppl 1:36-38.
35. Maitland GD. *Vertebral Manipulation.* 6th ed. London: Butterworths; 1986.
36. Busch AJ, Barber KA, Overend TJ, Peloso PM, Schachter CL. Exercise for treating fibromyalgia syndrome. *Cochrane Database Syst Rev.* 2007(4):CD003786.
37. Kuphal KE, Fibuch EE, Taylor BK. Extended swimming exercise reduces inflammatory and peripheral neuropathic pain in rodents. *J Pain.* Dec 2007;8(12):989-997.
38. Hoffman MD, Shepanski MA, Mackenzie SP, Clifford PS. Experimentally induced pain perception is acutely reduced by aerobic exercise in people with chronic low back pain. *J Rehabil Res Dev.* Mar-Apr 2005;42(2):183-190.
39. Butler D, Moseley G. *Explain Pain.* Adelaide: Noigroup; 2003.
40. Louw A, Puentedura EL, Mintken P. Use of an abbreviated neuroscience education approach in the treatment of chronic low back pain: a case report. *Physiotherapy theory and practice.* Jan 2012;28(1):50-62.
41. Barnard N. *Foods That Fight Pain.* New York: Three Rivers Press; 1998.
42. Wall PD, Melzack R. *Textbook of Pain.* 5th ed. London: Elsevier; 2005.
43. Wiendels NJ, Knuistingh Neven A, Rosendaal FR, et al. Chronic frequent headache in the general population: prevalence and associated factors. *Cephalalgia.* Dec 2006;26(12):1434-1442.

More patient books by Adriaan Louw

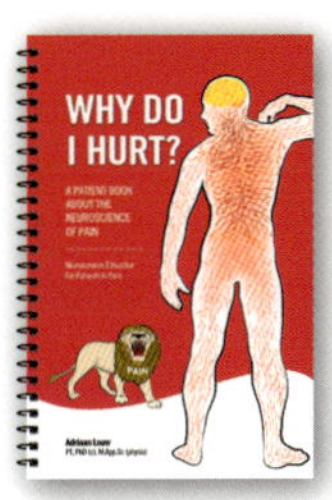

Why Do I Hurt?: A Patient Book About the Neuroscience of Pain

Pain is normal — living in pain is not. Learn the neuroscience behind your chronic pain — what pain really is — and take a big step toward living without it.

ITEM #8746

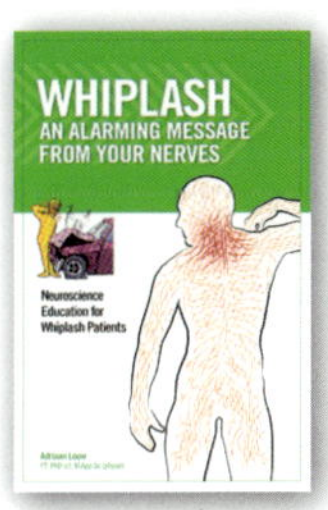

Whiplash: An Alarming Message from Your Nerves

Learn how your nerves become sensitive after a whiplash injury, how to ease the pain and why early, gentle movement is important for recovery.

ITEM #8744

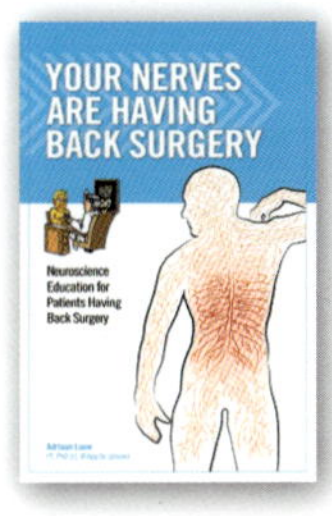

Your Nerves Are Having Back Surgery

Discover what your nervous system experiences when you undergo back surgery — why nerve sensitization occurs and how you can calm it down.

ITEM #8745

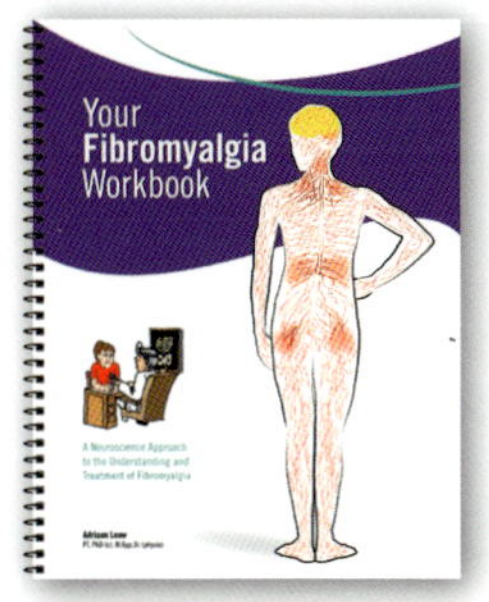

Your Fibromyalgia Workbook

Turn down your extra-sensitive nervous system. Understanding your pain lets you hurt less, do more and recover from fibromyalgia symptoms.

ITEM #8747

Therapeutic Neuroscience Education

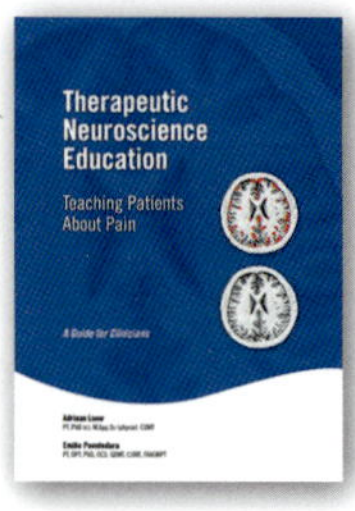

Medical professionals, educators and students, discover how neuroscience education can treat patients with chronic pain in Adriaan Louw and Emilio Puentedura's 304-page textbook *Therapeutic Neuroscience Education: Teaching Patients About Pain; A Guide for Clinicians.*

With roughly a quarter of the population living with chronic pain, clinicians are finding current diagnosis and treatment models to be increasingly inadequate. In order for movement-based therapy to be truly effective, you must first change the patients' faulty cognitions regarding their pain. Studies show that by educating the patient on what pain is and how it works, they experience less pain, are less fearful, move and exercise more, and are more willing to participate in therapy.

Physical therapists Louw and Puentedura deliver an evidence-based perspective on how the body and brain work together to create pain, teach how to convey this new view of pain to patients in a way that's easily understood and internalized, and demonstrate how to successfully integrate therapeutic neuroscience education into a practice.

ITEM #8748